METABOLIC RESET DIET FOR SENIORS

A Complete Guide for Senior Weight Loss, Energy, Hormonal Balance, Sexual Health and Longevity

Andrew H. Steve

About the Author

Andrew H. Steve, a renowned nutrition and health expert, specializes in empowering individuals over 40 to reclaim their health. With a passion for nutrition and a deep understanding of the human body and metabolism, Andrew has successfully guided many to achieve significant weight loss and enhanced well-being.

With over a decade of experience, Andrew's approach is far from one-size-fits-all. He tailors his advice to each individual, focusing on a holistic method that encompasses a balanced diet, mindful eating, and an active lifestyle, rather than just diets and restrictions.

Known for his ability to distill complex dietary concepts into practical, actionable strategies, Andrew is a guiding force in navigating the intricacies of metabolism and wellness. His dedication extends beyond his professional achievements, as he finds joy in outdoor activities, experimenting with new recipes, and engaging in healthy discussions.

If you're over 40 and looking to lose weight, increase energy, or improve your overall well-being, Andrew H. Steve is your ideal mentor. Under his guidance, you're not just adopting a healthy lifestyle; you're embarking on a transformative journey to rediscover your vitality and thrive.

TABLE OF CONTENTS

CHAPTER 1

INTRODUCTION

In the golden years of life, maintaining vitality and well-being becomes a cherished pursuit. Yet, as the sands of time trickle down, our bodies undergo profound changes, including shifts in metabolism that can significantly impact our health and quality of life. This journey into the realm of metabolic reset diets for seniors promises not just a glimpse but a comprehensive exploration into the art and science of rejuvenating one's metabolism to embrace a vibrant and fulfilling life.

Definition of Metabolic Reset Diet

Picture your metabolism as the engine that propels your body forward, converting fuel into energy and orchestrating a symphony of biochemical processes that keep you alive and thriving. However, as we age, this once-efficient engine may begin to sputter and falter, leading to a cascade of health challenges. Enter the metabolic reset diet, a beacon of hope amidst the tempest of metabolic slowdown.

But what exactly is a metabolic reset diet? In essence, it's a strategic dietary approach designed to recalibrate your metabolism, revitalize your energy levels, and reignite your zest for life. Unlike fad diets that promise quick fixes with questionable sustainability, a metabolic reset diet operates on the principles of nourishment, balance, and long-term health. It's about nurturing your body with the nutrients it needs to function optimally, while also addressing the unique metabolic challenges that accompany aging.

Importance of Nutrition for Seniors

Now, let's shine a spotlight on the cornerstone of vitality for seniors: nutrition. As the saying goes, "You are what you eat," and never is this truer than in the realm of senior health. Nutrition isn't just about filling your stomach; it's about fueling your body with the building blocks it needs to thrive, from the cellular level to the grand tapestry of your overall well-being.

For seniors, the importance of nutrition cannot be overstated. With each passing year, our bodies undergo a series of physiological changes that demand careful attention to dietary choices. From dwindling muscle mass to diminishing bone density, from fluctuating hormone levels to slower metabolic rates, the aging process presents a unique set of nutritional challenges.

But fear not, for the power of nutrition extends far beyond mere sustenance. It holds the key to unlocking vitality, resilience, and longevity. By embracing a diet rich in essential nutrients, seniors can bolster their immune systems, support healthy aging, and mitigate the risk of chronic diseases that often loom on the horizon.

Moreover, nutrition plays a pivotal role in enhancing cognitive function, mood stability, and overall mental well-being. As the brain's faithful steward, a well-nourished body lays the groundwork for sharp cognition, improved memory, and a sunny disposition that brightens even the gloomiest of days.

In essence, nutrition is the cornerstone upon which the edifice of senior health stands. It's the compass that guides us on our journey toward vitality and well-being, and it's the gentle hand that cradles us through the twists and turns of the aging process.

So, as we embark on this odyssey into the realm of metabolic reset diets for seniors, let us remember the profound importance of nourishing our bodies with intention, wisdom, and the boundless reservoir of love that fuels our journey through life.

Together, let's unravel the mysteries of metabolism, savor the richness of wholesome nutrition, and embrace the transformative power of a metabolic reset diet designed for the golden years. For in the dance of nourishment and rejuvenation, we discover the timeless melody of vitality that sings in harmony with the rhythm of life itself.

CHAPTER 2

UNDERSTANDING METABOLISM

In the intricate tapestry of human biology, metabolism stands as a central pillar, orchestrating the ceaseless dance of energy production and utilization within our bodies. This chapter delves deep into the labyrinthine pathways of metabolism, shedding light on its nuances, its ebbs and flows, and its profound impact on the health and well-being of seniors.

Overview of Metabolism

At its core, metabolism encompasses a complex network of biochemical processes that occur within living organisms to sustain life. It encompasses two primary facets:

1. **Anabolism:** This is the constructive phase of metabolism where smaller molecules are synthesized into larger, more complex ones. Think of it as akin to building blocks being assembled to construct a grand edifice. Anabolic processes require energy input and include activities such as protein synthesis, DNA replication, and cellular growth.

2. **Catabolism:** In contrast, catabolism involves the breakdown of larger molecules into smaller ones, releasing energy in the process. It's like deconstructing the edifice to release the stored energy within. Catabolic processes include activities such as digestion, cellular respiration, and the breakdown of glycogen into glucose for energy production.

Together, these two opposing yet complementary processes form the cornerstone of metabolism, ensuring a delicate equilibrium that sustains life's myriad functions.

Changes in Metabolism with Age

As the sands of time trickle down, our bodies undergo a series of physiological changes that inevitably leave their mark on our metabolism. While the metabolic rate—the rate at which the body expends energy to sustain basic physiological functions—varies from person to person, several key changes commonly occur with age:

1. **Decreased Basal Metabolic Rate (BMR):** Basal metabolic rate refers to the number of calories the body needs to maintain basic physiological functions while at rest. With age, BMR tends to decrease, primarily due to a decline in lean muscle mass and changes in hormone levels. This decline in BMR means that older adults may

require fewer calories to maintain their weight, making weight management a crucial consideration.

2. **Changes in Body Composition:** Aging is often accompanied by a shift in body composition, characterized by a decrease in muscle mass and an increase in body fat. This alteration in body composition can further contribute to a decline in metabolic rate, as muscle tissue is metabolically more active than fat tissue.

3. **Hormonal Changes:** Hormones play a pivotal role in regulating metabolism, and their levels can fluctuate with age. For example, a decline in estrogen and testosterone levels in postmenopausal women and aging men, respectively, can impact metabolism and body composition. Additionally, changes in thyroid function, insulin sensitivity, and other hormonal factors can influence metabolic processes.

4. **Reduced Physical Activity:** As we age, it's common for physical activity levels to decrease due to various factors such as mobility issues, chronic health conditions, or simply lifestyle changes. This reduction in physical activity can contribute to a decline in overall energy expenditure, further influencing metabolic rate.

5. **Altered Nutrient Utilization:** Aging can affect the body's ability to efficiently utilize nutrients, including carbohydrates, fats, and proteins. For example, insulin sensitivity may decrease with age, leading to impaired glucose metabolism and an increased risk of insulin resistance and type 2 diabetes. Similarly, changes in lipid metabolism and protein synthesis can also occur with age, impacting overall metabolic health.

Impact of Metabolic Changes on Seniors

The repercussions of age-related metabolic changes ripple through every facet of senior health and well-being, shaping the landscape of vitality and resilience in profound ways:

1. **Weight Management:** With a decrease in metabolic rate and changes in body composition, weight management becomes a pivotal concern for seniors. Maintaining a healthy weight not only supports overall well-being but also mitigates the risk of chronic diseases such as obesity, diabetes, and cardiovascular disorders.

2. **Energy Levels:** The decline in metabolic rate and alterations in nutrient utilization can impact energy levels, leaving seniors feeling fatigued and lethargic. Optimizing nutrition and lifestyle factors to support

metabolic health can help sustain energy levels and enhance overall vitality.

3. **Nutritional Requirements:** Age-related changes in metabolism can influence the body's nutritional requirements, necessitating adjustments in dietary intake to meet these changing needs. Adequate intake of essential nutrients such as protein, vitamins, and minerals becomes paramount for supporting metabolic health and overall well-being.

4. **Chronic Disease Risk:** Age-related metabolic changes can predispose seniors to an increased risk of chronic diseases such as obesity, diabetes, cardiovascular disorders, and metabolic syndrome. Addressing modifiable risk factors through lifestyle interventions, including diet and exercise, is crucial for mitigating these risks and promoting long-term health.

5. **Quality of Life:** The interplay between metabolism and overall health directly impacts the quality of life for seniors. By optimizing metabolic health through targeted interventions, seniors can enhance their vitality, resilience, and independence, fostering a fulfilling and enriching life as they age.

CHAPTER 3

PRINCIPLES OF THE METABOLIC RESET DIET

Welcome to the heart of the metabolic reset journey, where we delve into the foundational principles that underpin this transformative dietary approach. In this chapter, we'll explore the crucial pillars of balanced macronutrient intake, the importance of micronutrients, and the essential role of hydration in resetting your metabolism and reclaiming your vitality.

Balanced Macronutrient Intake

Let's kick off our exploration with a deep dive into the world of macronutrients – the building blocks of our dietary landscape. Macronutrients, commonly referred to as "macros," encompass three primary categories: carbohydrates, proteins, and fats. Each of these macronutrients plays a distinct role in fueling our bodies and supporting various physiological functions.

1. **Carbohydrates**: Often vilified in the realm of trendy diets, carbohydrates are, in fact, an essential source of energy for our bodies. Found in an array of foods ranging from fruits and vegetables to grains and legumes, carbohydrates provide the fuel needed to

power our daily activities and fuel our metabolic processes.

- **Complex vs. Simple Carbohydrates:** It's crucial to distinguish between complex carbohydrates, which are rich in fiber and digested slowly, providing sustained energy, and simple carbohydrates, which are quickly digested and can lead to rapid spikes in blood sugar levels.

- **The Glycemic Index:** Understanding the glycemic index (GI) of carbohydrates can help guide your food choices, with lower GI foods providing more stable energy levels and better metabolic control.

2. **Proteins**: Often hailed as the building blocks of life, proteins are integral to the growth, repair, and maintenance of tissues throughout the body. Found in foods such as meat, fish, poultry, eggs, dairy, legumes, and nuts, proteins are comprised of amino acids, which serve as the body's essential structural components.

- **Complete vs. Incomplete Proteins:** While animal sources of protein typically provide all essential amino acids, plant-based sources may require combination or supplementation to ensure a complete amino acid profile.

- **Protein Quality:** Assessing the quality of protein sources involves considering factors such as digestibility, amino acid composition, and bioavailability, all of which influence the body's ability to utilize protein for various physiological functions.

3. **Fats**: Despite their demonization in certain dietary circles, fats are vital for numerous physiological functions, including hormone production, cellular structure, and nutrient absorption. Found in foods such as avocados, nuts, seeds, olive oil, fatty fish, and coconut oil, healthy fats play a crucial role in supporting metabolic health and overall well-being.

- **Healthy vs. Unhealthy Fats:** Not all fats are created equal. While healthy fats like monounsaturated and polyunsaturated fats promote heart health and metabolic function, unhealthy trans fats and excessive saturated fats can contribute to inflammation and metabolic dysfunction.

- **Omega-3 Fatty Acids:** These essential fats, found primarily in fatty fish, flaxseeds, chia seeds, and walnuts, are renowned for their anti-inflammatory properties and their role in supporting cardiovascular health and cognitive function.

Achieving a balanced macronutrient intake involves striking the right balance between carbohydrates, proteins, and fats to support your body's unique metabolic needs and promote optimal health. By embracing a diverse array of whole foods and mindful portion control, you can harness the power of macronutrients to fuel your metabolic reset journey and unlock your full potential.

Importance of Micronutrients

Now, let's shift our focus to the often-overlooked yet equally essential realm of micronutrients – the vitamins, minerals, and antioxidants that serve as the unsung heroes of our dietary landscape. While macronutrients provide the energy needed to fuel our bodies, micronutrients play a critical role in supporting cellular function, immune health, and metabolic regulation.

1. **Vitamins**: These organic compounds play a diverse range of roles in the body, from supporting immune

function to promoting collagen synthesis and facilitating energy production. While a varied diet rich in fruits, vegetables, whole grains, and lean proteins can provide many essential vitamins, certain populations, including seniors, may benefit from supplementation to address specific nutrient needs.

- **Vitamin D:** Often referred to as the "sunshine vitamin," vitamin D plays a crucial role in calcium absorption, bone health, immune function, and mood regulation. Seniors, who may have limited sun exposure and reduced skin synthesis of vitamin D, are particularly vulnerable to deficiency and may require supplementation to maintain optimal levels.

- **Vitamin B12:** Essential for nerve function, DNA synthesis, and red blood cell production, vitamin B12 is primarily found in animal-derived foods such as meat, fish, eggs, and dairy. Seniors, especially those following plant-based diets or experiencing gastrointestinal issues that impair nutrient absorption, may require supplemental B12 to prevent deficiency.

2. **Minerals**: These inorganic elements are essential for numerous physiological processes, including bone

health, muscle function, and nerve transmission. While minerals like calcium, magnesium, and potassium are well-known for their roles in supporting overall health, others, such as zinc, selenium, and iron, are equally vital for immune function, antioxidant defence, and energy metabolism.

- **Calcium and Bone Health:** As we age, maintaining optimal bone density becomes increasingly crucial to prevent fractures and osteoporosis. Adequate calcium intake, along with vitamin D and weight-bearing exercise, plays a central role in supporting bone health and preventing age-related bone loss.

- **Magnesium and Muscle Function:** This essential mineral is involved in over 300 biochemical reactions in the body, including muscle contraction, nerve function, and energy metabolism. Seniors, who may be at increased risk of magnesium deficiency due to factors such as reduced dietary intake, medication use, and impaired absorption, can benefit from incorporating magnesium-rich foods like leafy greens, nuts, seeds, and whole grains into their diets.

3. **Antioxidants**: These powerful compounds play a vital role in protecting our cells from oxidative damage caused by free radicals, which are unstable molecules that can contribute to aging, inflammation, and chronic disease. Found in a variety of plant-based foods such as fruits, vegetables, nuts, seeds, and spices, antioxidants help neutralize free radicals and support overall health and longevity.

    - **Role of Antioxidants in Aging**: As we age, our bodies become more susceptible to oxidative stress, which can accelerate cellular aging and contribute to the development of age-related diseases such as cardiovascular disease, neurodegenerative disorders, and cancer. By incorporating antioxidant-rich foods into their diets, seniors can support cellular health, mitigate oxidative damage, and promote healthy aging.

    - **Key Antioxidants:** Some of the most well-known antioxidants include vitamins C and E, beta-carotene, flavonoids, and polyphenols, which are found in a variety of colorful fruits and vegetables, as well as herbs, spices, and teas.

By prioritizing a diet rich in a diverse array of colorful fruits and vegetables, whole grains, lean proteins, and healthy fats, seniors can ensure adequate intake of essential micronutrients to support cellular health, immune function, and metabolic regulation. Additionally, targeted supplementation may be beneficial for addressing specific nutrient needs and optimizing overall well-being.

Role of Hydration

Last but certainly not least, let's turn our attention to the unsung hero of metabolic health: hydration. While often overlooked in the realm of dietary priorities, proper hydration plays a pivotal role in supporting metabolic function, cognitive performance, and overall well-being.

1. **Water as a Vital Nutrient**: Water is not only essential for life but also serves as a fundamental nutrient that supports numerous physiological functions, including nutrient transport, temperature regulation, waste removal, and joint lubrication. Adequate hydration is crucial for maintaining optimal metabolic function, supporting cognitive performance, and promoting overall health and well-being.

2. **Hydration and Metabolism**: Dehydration can impair metabolic function and lead to a host of health

challenges, including fatigue, cognitive decline, and compromised immune function. Studies have shown that even mild dehydration can negatively impact metabolic rate and energy expenditure, highlighting the importance of prioritizing hydration for optimal metabolic health.

3. **Signs of Dehydration**: Recognizing the signs of dehydration is essential for maintaining optimal hydration status and supporting metabolic health. Common symptoms of dehydration include thirst, dry mouth, dark urine, fatigue, dizziness, and headaches. Seniors, who may have a diminished thirst sensation and reduced kidney function, are particularly vulnerable to dehydration and should pay close attention to their fluid intake.

4. **Hydration Recommendations**: While individual fluid needs vary based on factors such as age, gender, activity level, and climate, general guidelines recommend consuming approximately 8-10 cups (64-80 ounces) of fluid per day for adults, with additional fluid needed to replace losses from exercise, heat, or illness. Hydration needs may be higher for seniors, who may have decreased thirst sensation, reduced kidney function, and increased risk of dehydration.

5. **Sources of Hydration**: While water is the primary source of hydration, other beverages and foods can contribute to overall fluid intake. In addition to plain water, hydrating beverages such as herbal teas, infused water, coconut water, and diluted fruit juices can help meet fluid needs. Additionally, water-rich foods such as fruits, vegetables, soups, and broths can contribute to overall hydration.

CHAPTER 4

BENEFITS OF METABOLIC RESET DIET FOR SENIORS

In the symphony of life, the melody of vitality is composed of myriad harmonies, each playing a crucial role in orchestrating our well-being. As we delve into the realm of metabolic reset diets for seniors, we uncover a treasure trove of benefits that resonate deeply with the aspirations of those seeking to embrace the fullness of life. From weight management to sharpened mental acuity, from boundless energy to fortified defences against disease, the benefits of a metabolic reset diet weave a tapestry of rejuvenation and vitality for seniors.

Weight Management

Weight management stands as a cornerstone of health, especially as we age. The metabolic reset diet offers a beacon of hope for seniors navigating the complex landscape of weight fluctuations and stubborn pounds. By recalibrating the body's metabolic machinery, this dietary approach sets the stage for sustainable weight management that transcends the confines of mere numbers on a scale.

One of the primary mechanisms through which a metabolic reset diet supports weight management is by promoting a balanced intake of macronutrients. By prioritizing whole foods rich in essential nutrients and fiber while minimizing processed foods laden with empty calories, seniors can foster a sense of satiety and satisfaction that curbs overeating and snacking.

Moreover, the metabolic reset diet emphasizes portion control, encouraging seniors to tune in to their body's hunger and fullness cues rather than mindlessly consuming food. By fostering mindful eating practices, this dietary approach cultivates a deeper connection with one's body and its nutritional needs, paving the way for more intuitive and balanced eating habits.

Furthermore, the metabolic reset diet emphasizes hydration as a crucial component of weight management. By staying adequately hydrated, seniors can support their body's metabolic processes, enhance digestion, and stave off cravings often mistaken for hunger.

In essence, the metabolic reset diet offers seniors a roadmap to navigate the complexities of weight management with grace and efficacy. By embracing a balanced approach to nutrition, portion control, and hydration, seniors can reclaim agency over their health and embark on a journey toward sustainable weight management that honours the wisdom of their bodies.

Energy Levels

Vibrant energy pulses at the heart of a life well-lived, fueling our pursuits, passions, and adventures with boundless enthusiasm. Yet, as the years unfurl, the ebb and flow of energy may wane, leaving seniors yearning for the vitality that once coursed through their veins. Enter the metabolic reset diet, a beacon of light amidst the shadows of fatigue and lethargy.

One of the hallmark benefits of the metabolic reset diet for seniors is its profound impact on energy levels. By nourishing the body with a balanced array of macronutrients, micronutrients, and hydration, this dietary approach replenishes the body's energy stores and ignites a newfound zest for life.

Central to the metabolic reset diet's ability to bolster energy levels is its emphasis on whole, nutrient-dense foods that provide a steady stream of fuel to power the body's metabolic machinery. By prioritizing complex carbohydrates, lean proteins, healthy fats, and fiber-rich fruits and vegetables, seniors can sustainably fuel their bodies and banish the dreaded midday slump.

Moreover, the metabolic reset diet promotes hydration as a cornerstone of vibrant energy. By staying adequately hydrated, seniors can fend off dehydration-induced fatigue and maintain optimal cognitive and physical function throughout the day.

Furthermore, the metabolic reset diet encourages seniors to tune in to their body's hunger and fullness cues, fostering a more intuitive and balanced approach to eating that supports sustained energy levels. By practicing mindful eating and honoring their body's nutritional needs, seniors can unlock the boundless reservoir of energy that lies within.

In essence, the metabolic reset diet serves as a catalyst for revitalizing energy levels and reclaiming the vitality that propels seniors forward on their journey through life. By nourishing the body with intention, wisdom, and a deep respect for its innate wisdom, seniors can bask in the radiance of boundless energy and embrace each day with renewed vigor.

Mental Clarity

In the intricate tapestry of human experience, mental clarity shines as a beacon of lucidity, guiding our thoughts, decisions, and actions with precision and purpose. Yet, as the sands of time trickle down, the veil of mental fog may descend, obscuring our cognitive faculties and leaving seniors yearning for the clarity of mind that once illuminated their path. Enter the metabolic reset diet, a steadfast ally in the quest for sharpened mental acuity and cognitive vitality.

One of the profound benefits of the metabolic reset diet for seniors is its transformative impact on mental clarity. By nourishing the brain with a balanced array of nutrients, hydration, and mindful eating practices, this dietary approach unfurls the fog of mental fatigue and revitalizes cognitive function with newfound clarity and focus.

Central to the metabolic reset diet's ability to enhance mental clarity is its emphasis on whole, nutrient-dense foods that fuel the brain's intricate network of neurons and neurotransmitters. By prioritizing foods rich in omega-3 fatty acids, antioxidants, vitamins, and minerals, seniors can nourish their brains and support optimal cognitive function.

Moreover, the metabolic reset diet champions hydration as a cornerstone of mental clarity. By staying adequately hydrated, seniors can fend off dehydration-induced brain fog and maintain optimal cognitive function throughout the day.

Furthermore, the metabolic reset diet encourages seniors to cultivate mindfulness in their eating habits, tuning in to their body's hunger and fullness cues and savoring each bite with intention and presence. By practicing mindful eating, seniors can foster a deeper connection with their food and its impact on their mental well-being.

In essence, the metabolic reset diet serves as a catalyst for sharpening mental acuity and reclaiming the clarity of mind that illuminates our path through life's myriad adventures. By nourishing the brain with wisdom, intention, and a deep reverence for its miraculous capabilities, seniors can bask in the brilliance of mental clarity and embrace each moment with renewed vigor.

Disease Prevention

In the grand tapestry of life, the specter of disease looms as a formidable adversary, threatening to derail our journey toward health and vitality. Yet, armed with the transformative power of nutrition, seniors can fortify their defenses and cultivate resilience in the face of illness. Enter the metabolic reset diet, a potent ally in the battle against chronic disease and a steadfast guardian of well-being.

One of the pivotal benefits of the metabolic reset diet for seniors is its profound impact on disease prevention. By nourishing the body with a balanced array of nutrients, antioxidants, and anti-inflammatory foods, this dietary approach strengthens the body's immune system and bolsters its defenses against a myriad of ailments.

Central to the metabolic reset diet's ability to prevent disease is its emphasis on whole, nutrient-dense foods that promote optimal immune function and combat inflammation. By prioritizing fruits, vegetables, lean proteins, healthy fats, and whole grains, seniors can arm their bodies with the nutritional ammunition needed to fend off illness and thrive in the face of adversity.

Moreover, the metabolic reset diet champions hydration as a cornerstone of disease prevention. By staying adequately hydrated, seniors can support optimal immune function, enhance detoxification pathways, and maintain the body's natural defenses against pathogens and toxins.

Furthermore, the metabolic reset diet encourages seniors to adopt lifestyle habits that promote overall well-being, such as regular physical activity, stress management techniques, and adequate sleep. By cultivating a holistic approach to health, seniors can create a fortified fortress of resilience that withstands the test of time and guards against the onslaught of disease.

In essence, the metabolic reset diet stands as a beacon of hope in the fight against chronic disease, offering seniors a pathway to vitality, resilience, and well-being. By nourishing the body with intention, wisdom, and a deep reverence for its innate healing capabilities, seniors can fortify their defenses and embrace a life of vibrant health and vitality.

As we journey through the myriad benefits of the metabolic reset diet for seniors, we uncover a treasure trove of rejuvenation and vitality that beckons us forward on the path to optimal health and well-being. From weight management to energy levels, mental clarity to disease prevention, the transformative power of nutrition holds the key to unlocking the boundless potential that resides within each and every one of us. So, let us embark on this odyssey with open hearts and minds, embracing the wisdom of the ages and the transformative power of a metabolic reset diet designed to nourish our bodies, minds, and spirits with intention, wisdom, and boundless love

CHAPTER 5

KEY COMPONENTS OF THE METABOLIC RESET DIET

In our quest for vitality and well-being, the foundation of a metabolic reset diet rests upon the pillars of mindful nourishment, balanced choices, and a deep understanding of the foods that fuel our bodies. As we delve into the key components of this transformative dietary approach, let us embark on a journey of exploration, discovery, and empowerment.

Whole Foods vs. Processed Foods

At the heart of the metabolic reset diet lies a fundamental choice: whole foods or processed foods? It's a choice that transcends mere sustenance, for it shapes the very landscape of our health and vitality.

Whole foods, in their pristine, unadulterated state, are gifts from nature's bounty. They are the vibrant fruits and vegetables that burst with colour and vitality, the nourishing grains and legumes that anchor our meals with wholesome sustenance, and the lean proteins that fuel our muscles and fortify our bodies.

In contrast, processed foods bear the mark of human intervention, transformed through a myriad of chemical processes, preservatives, and additives. They are the packaged snacks that tempt us from grocery store shelves, the sugary beverages that seduce our taste buds, and the convenience foods that promise quick fixes at the expense of our well-being.

But why does this choice matter, you may ask? The answer lies in the profound impact that whole foods and processed foods wield upon our bodies, from the cellular level to the grand tapestry of our overall health.

Whole foods, rich in vitamins, minerals, and phytonutrients, offer a symphony of health benefits that nourish our bodies from the inside out. They provide the raw materials our cells need to thrive, support optimal organ function, and promote a robust immune system that wards off illness and disease.

Moreover, whole foods boast a symphony of flavors and textures that awaken our senses and elevate the dining experience to a joyful celebration of nourishment and vitality. From the crisp crunch of an apple to the creamy richness of avocado, each bite is a testament to the abundant bounty of nature's harvest.

On the other hand, processed foods, laden with refined sugars, unhealthy fats, and artificial additives, wreak havoc on our bodies in ways both subtle and profound. They spike our blood sugar levels, wreak havoc on our hormonal balance, and contribute to a host of chronic diseases, from obesity and diabetes to heart disease and cancer.

Yet, in a world inundated with processed foods masquerading as quick fixes and convenient solutions, navigating the terrain of whole foods can seem like a daunting task. But fear not, for the journey toward vibrant health begins with a single step, a simple choice to prioritize whole, nutrient-dense foods that nourish our bodies and nurture our well-being.

Importance of Fiber

In the intricate tapestry of nutrition, fiber stands as a silent hero, an unsung champion of digestive health, metabolic balance, and overall well-being. Yet, despite its myriad benefits, fiber often remains an overlooked and underappreciated component of the modern diet.

But what exactly is fiber, and why is it so crucial for our health? Simply put, fiber is the indigestible portion of plant-based foods that passes through our digestive system relatively intact. It comes in two primary forms: soluble fiber, which dissolves in water to form a gel-like substance, and insoluble fiber, which adds bulk to our stool and aids in bowel regularity.

From regulating blood sugar levels to promoting healthy cholesterol levels, fiber plays a pivotal role in maintaining metabolic balance and warding off chronic diseases. It acts as a natural appetite suppressant, helping us feel fuller for longer and curbing cravings that can lead to overeating and weight gain.

Moreover, fiber serves as a prebiotic, nourishing the beneficial bacteria in our gut microbiome and supporting optimal digestive function. A healthy gut microbiome is crucial for nutrient absorption, immune function, and even mood regulation, underscoring the far-reaching impact of fiber on our overall well-being.

Yet, despite its myriad benefits, many individuals fall short of meeting their daily fiber needs, often due to the prevalence of processed foods that are stripped of this vital nutrient. But fear not, for incorporating fiber-rich foods into your diet is simpler than you may think.

From fruits and vegetables to whole grains and legumes, a diverse array of plant-based foods offer a rich tapestry of flavors and textures that make meeting your fiber needs a delicious and enjoyable endeavor. So, embrace the abundance of nature's bounty, and let fiber be your steadfast companion on the journey toward vibrant health and well-being.

Managing Portion Sizes

In a world of super-sized meals and bottomless buffets, managing portion sizes can seem like a Herculean task. Yet, in the realm of the metabolic reset diet, mastering the art of portion control is a cornerstone of success, empowering you to nourish your body with intention, balance, and mindfulness.

But why is portion control so crucial, you may wonder? The answer lies in the delicate balance between energy intake and expenditure, a dance of calories consumed and calories burned that ultimately determines our weight and metabolic health.

In an era where oversized portions have become the norm, it's all too easy to lose sight of what constitutes a balanced meal. Yet, by tuning into your body's hunger and satiety cues, you can cultivate a deeper awareness of portion sizes that support your health goals and promote metabolic balance.

So, how can you navigate the terrain of portion control with confidence and ease? It begins with a simple shift in mindset, from viewing food as mere fuel to embracing it as a source of nourishment, pleasure, and vitality.

Start by listening to your body's hunger signals and honoring its cues of satiety. Rather than mindlessly devouring large portions in a single sitting, savor each bite mindfully, chewing slowly and savoring the flavors and textures of your meal.

Moreover, be mindful of portion sizes when dining out or preparing meals at home. Opt for smaller plates and bowls to naturally limit portion sizes, and be mindful of serving sizes when plating your meals. Remember, it's not about deprivation or restriction but rather about finding a balanced approach that honors your body's needs and supports your health goals.

By mastering the art of portion control, you can nourish your body with the right amount of food to support your energy needs, promote metabolic balance, and embark on a journey toward vibrant health and well-being

CHAPTER 6

Breakfast Recipes

1. Avocado and Egg Breakfast Bowl

Ingredients:

- 1 ripe avocado

- 2 eggs

- ½ cup cherry tomatoes, halved

- ¼ cup diced red onion

- 1 tablespoon chopped cilantro

- Salt and pepper to taste

Instructions:

1. Cut the avocado in half and remove the pit. Scoop out a bit of flesh from each half to make room for the eggs.

2. Crack an egg into each avocado half.

3. Place the avocado halves on a baking sheet lined with parchment paper.

4. Surround the avocado halves with cherry tomatoes and sprinkle diced red onion over the top.

5. Season with salt and pepper.

6. Bake at 375°F (190°C) for 12-15 minutes or until the egg whites are set but the yolks are still runny.

7. Garnish with chopped cilantro before serving.

Nutritional Information (per serving):

- Calories: 310 kcal

- Protein: 11g

- Carbohydrates: 15g

- Fat: 24g

- Fiber: 10g

2. Greek Yogurt Parfait

Ingredients:

- 1 cup Greek yogurt

- ½ cup mixed berries (such as strawberries, blueberries, and raspberries)

- ¼ cup granola

- 1 tablespoon honey (optional)

Instructions:

1. In a serving glass or bowl, layer Greek yogurt, mixed berries, and granola.

2. Repeat the layers until all ingredients are used.

3. Drizzle honey on top if desired.

4. Serve immediately.

Nutritional Information (per serving):

- Calories: 280 kcal

- Protein: 18g

- Carbohydrates: 35g

- Fat: 7g

- Fiber: 5g

3. Spinach and Feta Omelette

Ingredients:

- 2 eggs

- 1 cup fresh spinach leaves

- 2 tablespoons crumbled feta cheese

- ¼ cup diced tomatoes

- Salt and pepper to taste

- Cooking spray or olive oil for greasing the pan

Instructions:

1. In a bowl, whisk the eggs until well beaten.

2. Heat a non-stick skillet over medium heat and lightly grease with cooking spray or olive oil.

3. Add the spinach leaves to the skillet and cook until wilted.

4. Pour the beaten eggs over the spinach.

5. Sprinkle crumbled feta cheese and diced tomatoes over the eggs.

6. Season with salt and pepper.

7. Cook until the edges of the omelette start to set, then gently fold it in half.

8. Continue cooking until the omelette is cooked through.

9. Transfer to a plate and serve hot.

Nutritional Information (per serving):

- Calories: 220 kcal

- Protein: 18g

- Carbohydrates: 4g

- Fat: 15g

- Fiber: 1g

4. Quinoa Breakfast Bowl

Ingredients:

- ½ cup cooked quinoa

- ¼ cup sliced almonds

- ¼ cup diced apples

- 1 tablespoon honey

- ½ teaspoon cinnamon

- ¼ cup Greek yogurt

Instructions:

1. In a bowl, combine cooked quinoa, sliced almonds, diced apples, honey, and cinnamon.

2. Mix well to combine.

3. Top with Greek yogurt before serving.

Nutritional Information (per serving):

- Calories: 300 kcal

- Protein: 11g

- Carbohydrates: 40g

- Fat: 12g

- Fiber: 6g

5. Chia Seed Pudding

Ingredients:

- 2 tablespoons chia seeds

- ½ cup unsweetened almond milk

- ¼ teaspoon vanilla extract

- ½ cup mixed berries (such as strawberries, blueberries, and raspberries)

- 1 tablespoon chopped nuts (such as almonds or walnuts)

- 1 teaspoon honey (optional)

Instructions:

1. In a bowl, combine chia seeds, almond milk, and vanilla extract.

2. Stir well and let it sit for at least 30 minutes or overnight in the refrigerator until it thickens.

3. Once the chia seed pudding has thickened, layer it in a serving glass or bowl with mixed berries and chopped nuts.

4. Drizzle honey on top if desired.

5. Serve chilled.

Nutritional Information (per serving):

- Calories: 240 kcal

- Protein: 7g

- Carbohydrates: 27g

- Fat: 13g

- Fiber: 12g

6. Smoked Salmon and Avocado Toast

Ingredients:

- 1 slice whole grain bread, toasted

- 2 ounces smoked salmon

- 1/4 ripe avocado, sliced

- 1 tablespoon capers

- 1 teaspoon lemon juice

- Fresh dill for garnish

Instructions:

1. Top the toasted whole grain bread with sliced smoked salmon.

2. Arrange avocado slices on top of the salmon.

3. Sprinkle capers over the avocado slices.

4. Drizzle lemon juice over the toast.

5. Garnish with fresh dill before serving.

Nutritional Information (per serving):

- Calories: 250 kcal

- Protein: 16g

- Carbohydrates: 14g

- Fat: 15g

- Fiber: 5g

7. Veggie and Cheese Breakfast Wrap

Ingredients:

- 1 whole grain tortilla

- 2 eggs, scrambled

- ¼ cup diced bell peppers (any color)

- ¼ cup diced onions

- ¼ cup shredded cheddar cheese

- Salt and pepper to taste

- Cooking spray or olive oil for greasing the pan

Instructions:

1. Heat a non-stick skillet over medium heat and lightly grease with cooking spray or olive oil.

2. Add diced bell peppers and onions to the skillet and cook until softened.

3. Add scrambled eggs to the skillet and cook until set.

4. Warm the whole grain tortilla in the skillet or microwave.

5. Place the scrambled eggs, cooked bell peppers, onions, and shredded cheddar cheese on the tortilla.

6. Season with salt and pepper.

7. Roll up the tortilla to form a wrap.

8. Serve warm.

Nutritional Information (per serving):

- Calories: 330 kcal

* Protein: 20g

* Carbohydrates: 24g

* Fat: 17g

* Fiber: 5g

8. Berry and Almond Butter Smoothie

Ingredients:

* 1 cup unsweetened almond milk

* 1/2 cup mixed berries (such as strawberries, blueberries, and raspberries)

* 1 tablespoon almond butter

* 1 tablespoon chia seeds

* 1 teaspoon honey (optional)

* Ice cubes (optional)

Instructions:

1. In a blender, combine almond milk, mixed berries, almond butter, chia seeds, and honey.

2. Blend until smooth.

3. Add ice cubes if desired and blend again until well combined.

4. Pour the smoothie into a glass and serve immediately.

Nutritional Information (per serving):

- Calories: 250 kcal

- Protein: 7g

- Carbohydrates: 20g

- Fat: 16g

- Fiber: 8g

Lunch Recipes

1. Mediterranean Chickpea Salad

Ingredients:

- 1 can (15 ounces) chickpeas, drained and rinsed

- 1 cup cherry tomatoes, halved

- 1 cucumber, diced

- ¼ cup diced red onion

- ¼ cup chopped fresh parsley

- 2 tablespoons extra virgin olive oil

- 1 tablespoon lemon juice

- 1 teaspoon dried oregano

- Salt and pepper to taste

- Crumbled feta cheese (optional)

Instructions:

1. In a large bowl, combine chickpeas, cherry tomatoes, cucumber, red onion, and parsley.

2. Drizzle extra virgin olive oil and lemon juice over the salad.

3. Sprinkle dried oregano, salt, and pepper.

4. Toss until well combined.

5. Top with crumbled feta cheese if desired.

6. Serve chilled.

Nutritional Information (per serving):

- Calories: 280 kcal

- Protein: 10g

- Carbohydrates: 30g

- Fat: 14g

- Fiber: 9g

2. Grilled Chicken and Vegetable Skewers

Ingredients:

- 2 boneless, skinless chicken breasts, cut into cubes

- 1 bell pepper, cut into chunks

- 1 zucchini, sliced into rounds

- 1 yellow squash, sliced into rounds

- 1 red onion, cut into chunks

- 2 tablespoons olive oil

- 1 teaspoon dried Italian seasoning

- Salt and pepper to taste

Instructions:

1. Preheat the grill to medium-high heat.

2. Thread chicken cubes and vegetables onto skewers.

3. Drizzle olive oil over the skewers and sprinkle with dried Italian seasoning, salt, and pepper.

4. Grill the skewers for 8-10 minutes, turning occasionally, until the chicken is cooked through and the vegetables are tender.

5. Serve hot.

Nutritional Information (per serving):

- Calories: 320 kcal

- Protein: 28g

- Carbohydrates: 10g

- Fat: 18g

- Fiber: 3g

3. Quinoa and Black Bean Stuffed Bell Peppers

Ingredients:

- 4 bell peppers, halved and seeds removed

- 1 cup cooked quinoa

- 1 can (15 ounces) black beans, drained and rinsed

- 1 cup corn kernels (fresh or frozen)

- 1 cup diced tomatoes

- ½ cup shredded cheddar cheese

- 1 teaspoon chili powder

- ½ teaspoon cumin

- Salt and pepper to taste

Instructions:

1. Preheat the oven to 375°F (190°C).

2. In a large bowl, combine cooked quinoa, black beans, corn kernels, diced tomatoes, shredded cheddar cheese, chili powder, cumin, salt, and pepper.

3. Spoon the quinoa mixture into the halved bell peppers.

4. Place the stuffed bell peppers in a baking dish.

5. Cover the dish with foil and bake for 25-30 minutes, or until the peppers are tender.

6. Remove the foil and bake for an additional 5 minutes to melt the cheese.

7. Serve hot.

Nutritional Information (per serving):

- Calories: 270 kcal

- Protein: 12g

- Carbohydrates: 38g

- Fat: 8g

- Fiber: 10g

4. Salmon and Asparagus Foil Packets

Ingredients:

- 2 salmon fillets

- 1 bunch asparagus, trimmed

- 2 tablespoons olive oil

- 2 cloves garlic, minced

- 1 lemon, sliced

- Salt and pepper to taste

Instructions:

1. Preheat the oven to 400°F (200°C).

2. Place each salmon fillet on a piece of aluminum foil large enough to fold into a packet.

3. Arrange asparagus spears around each salmon fillet.

4. Drizzle olive oil over the salmon and asparagus.

5. Sprinkle minced garlic over the top.

6. Place lemon slices on top of the salmon.

7. Season with salt and pepper.

8. Fold the foil over the salmon and asparagus to create a packet, sealing the edges tightly.

9. Place the foil packets on a baking sheet and bake for 15-20 minutes, or until the salmon is cooked through and the asparagus is tender.

10. Serve hot.

Nutritional Information (per serving):

- Calories: 320 kcal

- Protein: 28g

- Carbohydrates: 6g

- Fat: 20g

- Fiber: 3g

5. Turkey and Hummus Wrap

Ingredients:

- 1 whole grain tortilla

- 3 ounces sliced turkey breast

- 2 tablespoons hummus

- ¼ cup shredded lettuce

- ¼ cup sliced cucumber

- ¼ cup shredded carrots

- Salt and pepper to taste

Instructions:

1. Lay the whole grain tortilla flat on a clean surface.

2. Spread hummus evenly over the tortilla.

3. Layer sliced turkey breast, shredded lettuce, sliced cucumber, and shredded carrots on top of the hummus.

4. Season with salt and pepper.

5. Roll up the tortilla to form a wrap.

6. Slice the wrap in half and serve.

Nutritional Information (per serving):

- Calories: 270 kcal

- Protein: 20g

- Carbohydrates: 28g

- Fat: 10g

- Fiber: 6g

1. Baked Lemon Herb Chicken

Ingredients:

- 2 boneless, skinless chicken breasts
- 2 tablespoons olive oil
- 1 tablespoon lemon juice
- 1 teaspoon dried rosemary
- 1 teaspoon dried thyme
- 1 teaspoon dried parsley
- Salt and pepper to taste

Instructions:

1. Preheat the oven to 375°F (190°C).
2. In a small bowl, mix together olive oil, lemon juice, dried rosemary, dried thyme, dried parsley, salt, and pepper.
3. Place chicken breasts in a baking dish and brush with the herb mixture.
4. Bake for 25-30 minutes or until chicken is cooked through.

5. Serve hot with your choice of side dishes.

Nutritional Information (per serving):

- Calories: 280 kcal

- Protein: 30g

- Carbohydrates: 0g

- Fat: 17g

- Fiber: 0g

2. Veggie Stir-Fry with Tofu

Ingredients:

- 1 block (14 ounces) firm tofu, drained and cubed

- 2 cups mixed vegetables (such as bell peppers, broccoli, carrots, and snap peas)

- 2 tablespoons low-sodium soy sauce

- 1 tablespoon sesame oil

- 1 teaspoon minced garlic

- 1 teaspoon minced ginger

- Salt and pepper to taste

Instructions:

1. Heat sesame oil in a large skillet or wok over medium-high heat.

2. Add cubed tofu and cook until golden brown on all sides.

3. Add mixed vegetables, minced garlic, and minced ginger to the skillet.

4. Stir-fry for 5-7 minutes or until vegetables are tender-crisp.

5. Drizzle low-sodium soy sauce over the stir-fry and toss to combine.

6. Season with salt and pepper.

7. Serve hot over cooked brown rice or quinoa.

Nutritional Information (per serving):

- Calories: 320 kcal

- Protein: 20g

- Carbohydrates: 20g

- Fat: 18g

- Fiber: 6g

3. Lentil and Vegetable Soup

Ingredients:

- 1 cup dried green lentils

- 4 cups low-sodium vegetable broth

- 1 cup diced carrots

- 1 cup diced celery

- 1 cup diced onion

- 2 cloves garlic, minced

- 1 teaspoon dried thyme

- 1 teaspoon dried rosemary

- Salt and pepper to taste

Instructions:

1. Rinse lentils under cold water and drain.

2. In a large pot, combine lentils, vegetable broth, diced carrots, diced celery, diced onion, minced garlic, dried thyme, and dried rosemary.

3. Bring to a boil, then reduce heat and simmer for 25-30 minutes or until lentils and vegetables are tender.

4. Season with salt and pepper to taste.

5. Serve hot with a slice of whole grain bread.

Nutritional Information (per serving):

- Calories: 280 kcal

- Protein: 18g

- Carbohydrates: 48g

- Fat: 1g

- Fiber: 17g

4. Shrimp and Vegetable Stir-Fry

Ingredients:

- 8 ounces shrimp, peeled and deveined

- 2 cups mixed vegetables (such as bell peppers, broccoli, carrots, and snap peas)

- 2 tablespoons low-sodium soy sauce

- 1 tablespoon olive oil

- 1 teaspoon minced garlic

- Salt and pepper to taste

Instructions:

1. Heat olive oil in a large skillet or wok over medium-high heat.

2. Add shrimp to the skillet and cook until pink and opaque, about 2-3 minutes per side.

3. Remove shrimp from the skillet and set aside.

4. In the same skillet, add mixed vegetables and minced garlic.

5. Stir-fry for 5-7 minutes or until vegetables are tender-crisp.

6. Return shrimp to the skillet and drizzle low-sodium soy sauce over the stir-fry.

7. Toss to combine and season with salt and pepper.

8. Serve hot over cooked brown rice or quinoa.

Nutritional Information (per serving):

- Calories: 260 kcal

- Protein: 28g

- Carbohydrates: 20g

- Fat: 8g

- Fiber: 4g

5. Baked Salmon with Roasted Vegetables

Ingredients:

- 2 salmon fillets

- 2 cups mixed vegetables (such as bell peppers, zucchini, cherry tomatoes, and red onion)

- 2 tablespoons olive oil

- 1 teaspoon dried Italian seasoning

- Salt and pepper to taste

Instructions:

1. Preheat the oven to 400°F (200°C).

2. Place salmon fillets on a baking sheet lined with parchment paper.

3. In a bowl, toss mixed vegetables with olive oil, dried Italian seasoning, salt, and pepper.

4. Arrange the seasoned vegetables around the salmon fillets on the baking sheet.

5. Bake for 15-20 minutes or until salmon is cooked through and vegetables are tender.

6. Serve hot.

Nutritional Information (per serving):

- Calories: 300 kcal

- Protein: 24g

- Carbohydrates: 10g

- Fat: 18g

- Fiber: 4g

6. Turkey and Vegetable Skillet

Ingredients:

- 1pound ground turkey

- 2 cups mixed vegetables (such as bell peppers, zucchini, carrots, and spinach)

- 1 onion, diced

- 2 cloves garlic, minced

- 1 tablespoon olive oil

- 1 teaspoon dried Italian seasoning

- Salt and pepper to taste

Instructions:

1. Heat olive oil in a large skillet over medium heat.

2. Add diced onion and minced garlic to the skillet and sauté until softened.

3. Add ground turkey to the skillet and cook until browned.

4. Stir in mixed vegetables and dried Italian seasoning.

5. Cook for 5-7 minutes or until vegetables are tender.

6. Season with salt and pepper to taste.

7. Serve hot.

Nutritional Information (per serving):

- Calories: 290 kcal

- Protein: 25g

- Carbohydrates: 10g

- Fat: 15g

- Fiber: 3g

7. Eggplant Parmesan

Ingredients:

- 1 large eggplant, sliced into rounds

- 1 cup marinara sauce

- 1 cup shredded mozzarella cheese

- ¼ cup grated Parmesan cheese

- 2 tablespoons olive oil

- 1 teaspoon dried Italian seasoning

- Salt and pepper to taste

Instructions:

1. Preheat the oven to 375°F (190°C).

2. Brush both sides of eggplant slices with olive oil and season with dried Italian seasoning, salt, and pepper.

3. Place eggplant slices on a baking sheet lined with parchment paper.

4. Bake for 15-20 minutes or until tender.

5. Remove from the oven and spread marinara sauce over each eggplant slice.

6. Sprinkle shredded mozzarella cheese and grated Parmesan cheese over the sauce.

7. Return to the oven and bake for an additional 10-15 minutes or until cheese is melted and bubbly.

8. Serve hot.

Nutritional Information (per serving):

- Calories: 280 kcal

- Protein: 12g

- Carbohydrates: 15g

- Fat: 18g

- Fiber: 7g

8. Quinoa Stuffed Bell Peppers

Ingredients:

- 4 bell peppers, halved and seeds removed

- 1 cup cooked quinoa

- 1 cup black beans, drained and rinsed

- 1 cup diced tomatoes

- ½ cup shredded cheddar cheese

- 1 teaspoon chili powder

- ½ teaspoon cumin

- Salt and pepper to taste

Instructions:

1. Preheat the oven to 375°F (190°C).

2. In a large bowl, combine cooked quinoa, black beans, diced tomatoes, shredded cheddar cheese, chili powder, cumin, salt, and pepper.

3. Spoon the quinoa mixture into the halved bell peppers.

4. Place the stuffed bell peppers in a baking dish.

5. Cover the dish with foil and bake for 25-30 minutes, or until the peppers are tender.

6. Remove the foil and bake for an additional 5 minutes to melt the cheese.

7. Serve hot.

Nutritional Information (per serving):

- Calories: 270 kcal

- Protein: 14g

- Carbohydrates: 35g

- Fat: 8g

- Fiber: 8g

1. Baked Apple with Cinnamon

Ingredients:

- 1 large apple, cored and sliced
- 1 teaspoon cinnamon
- 1 teaspoon honey (optional)
- 1 tablespoon chopped walnuts (optional)

Instructions:

1. Preheat the oven to 375°F (190°C).
2. Place the apple slices in a baking dish.
3. Sprinkle cinnamon over the apple slices.
4. Drizzle honey over the apples if desired.
5. Bake for 15-20 minutes or until apples are tender.
6. Sprinkle chopped walnuts over the baked apples before serving.

Nutritional Information (per serving):

- Calories: 90 kcal
- Protein: 1g
- Carbohydrates: 20g

- Fat: 2g

- Fiber: 4g

2. Banana and Peanut Butter Bites

Ingredients:

- 1 banana, sliced

- 2 tablespoons natural peanut butter

- 2 tablespoons chopped dark chocolate or chocolate chips (optional)

Instructions:

1. Spread peanut butter on banana slices.

2. Sandwich two banana slices together to form bites.

3. Optionally, dip one side of the banana bites in chopped dark chocolate or chocolate chips.

4. Place the banana bites on a plate and freeze for 30 minutes before serving.

Nutritional Information (per serving):

- Calories: 150 kcal

- Protein: 3g

- Carbohydrates: 17g

- Fat: 8g

- Fiber: 3g

3. Greek Yogurt with Berries

Ingredients:

- ½ cup Greek yogurt

- ¼ cup mixed berries (such as strawberries, blueberries, and raspberries)

- 1 tablespoon honey (optional)

- 1 tablespoon sliced almonds (optional)

Instructions:

1. Spoon Greek yogurt into a serving bowl.

2. Top with mixed berries.

3. Drizzle honey over the yogurt and berries if desired.

4. Sprinkle sliced almonds over the top before serving.

Nutritional Information (per serving):

- Calories: 150 kcal

- Protein: 10g

- Carbohydrates: 18g

- Fat: 5g

- Fiber: 3g

4. Chia Seed Pudding with Mango

Ingredients:

- 2 tablespoons chia seeds

- ½ cup unsweetened almond milk

- ½ teaspoon vanilla extract

- ½ cup diced mango

- 1 tablespoon shredded coconut (optional)

- 1 teaspoon maple syrup (optional)

Instructions:

1. In a bowl, combine chia seeds, almond milk, and vanilla extract.

2. Stir well and let it sit for at least 30 minutes or overnight in the refrigerator until it thickens.

3. Once the chia seed pudding has thickened, layer it in a serving glass or bowl with diced mango.

4. Optionally, sprinkle shredded coconut over the pudding.

5. Optionally, drizzle maple syrup over the top before serving.

Nutritional Information (per serving):

- Calories: 200 kcal

- Protein: 6g

- Carbohydrates: 26g

- Fat: 8g

- Fiber: 9g

5. Baked Pear with Almonds

Ingredients:

- 1 ripe pear, halved and cored

- 1 tablespoon chopped almonds

- 1 teaspoon honey (optional)

- ¼ teaspoon cinnamon

Instructions:

1. Preheat the oven to 375°F (190°C).

2. Place the pear halves in a baking dish, cut side up.

3. Sprinkle chopped almonds over the pear halves.

4. Drizzle honey over the pears if desired.

5. Sprinkle cinnamon over the top.

6. Bake for 15-20 minutes or until pears are tender.

7. Serve hot.

Nutritional Information (per serving):

- Calories: 130 kcal

- Protein: 2g

- Carbohydrates: 23g

- Fat: 4g

- Fiber: 5g

6. Coconut Mango Rice Pudding

Ingredients:

- ½ cup cooked brown rice

- ½ cup coconut milk

- ½ cup diced mango

- 1 tablespoon shredded coconut

- 1 teaspoon maple syrup (optional)

- ¼ teaspoon vanilla extract

Instructions:

1. In a saucepan, combine cooked brown rice and coconut milk.

2. Cook over medium heat, stirring frequently, until thickened.

3. Stir in diced mango, shredded coconut, maple syrup (if using), and vanilla extract.

4. Cook for an additional 2-3 minutes.

5. Remove from heat and let it cool slightly before serving.

Nutritional Information (per serving):

- Calories: 180 kcal

- Protein: 2g

- Carbohydrates: 25g

- Fat: 8g

- Fiber: 3g

7. Almond Butter and Banana Ice Cream

Ingredients:

- 2 ripe bananas, peeled and sliced

- 2 tablespoons natural almond butter

- 1 tablespoon cocoa powder (optional)

- 1/4 teaspoon vanilla extract

Instructions:

1. Place sliced bananas in a single layer on a baking sheet lined with parchment paper.

2. Freeze for at least 2 hours or until solid.

3. In a food processor, combine frozen banana slices, almond butter, cocoa powder (if using), and vanilla extract.

4. Blend until smooth and creamy.

5. Serve immediately as soft-serve ice cream or transfer to a container and freeze for a firmer texture.

Nutritional Information (per serving):

- Calories: 220 kcal

- Protein: 4g

- Carbohydrates: 30g

- Fat: 10g

- Fiber: 4g

8. Berry and Yogurt Popsicles

Ingredients:

- 1 cup Greek yogurt

- 1/2 cup mixed berries (such as strawberries, blueberries, and raspberries)

- 1 tablespoon honey (optional)

Instructions:

1. In a blender, combine Greek yogurt, mixed berries, and honey (if using).

2. Blend until smooth.

3. Pour the mixture into popsicle molds.

4. Insert popsicle sticks into the molds.

5. Freeze for at least 4 hours or until solid.

6. Remove from molds and serve.

Nutritional Information (per serving):

- Calories: 70 kcal

- Protein: 5g

- Carbohydrates: 10g

- Fat: 1g

- Fiber: 1g

Sample Meal Plan

Day 1:

- Breakfast: Avocado and Egg Breakfast Bowl

- Lunch: Mediterranean Chickpea Salad

- Dinner: Baked Lemon Herb Chicken

- Dessert: Baked Apple with Cinnamon

Day 2:

- Breakfast: Greek Yogurt Parfait

- Lunch: Grilled Chicken and Vegetable Skewers

- Dinner: Lentil and Vegetable Soup

- Dessert: Banana and Peanut Butter Bites

Day 3:

- Breakfast: Spinach and Feta Omelette

- Lunch: Quinoa and Black Bean Stuffed Bell Peppers

- Dinner: Shrimp and Vegetable Stir-Fry

- Dessert: Greek Yogurt with Berries

Day 4:

- Breakfast: Quinoa Breakfast Bowl

- Lunch: Salmon and Asparagus Foil Packets

- Dinner: Turkey and Vegetable Skillet

- Dessert: Chia Seed Pudding with Mango

Day 5:

- Breakfast: Chia Seed Pudding

- Lunch: Eggplant Parmesan

- Dinner: Baked Salmon with Roasted Vegetables

- Dessert: Baked Pear with Almonds

Day 6:

- Breakfast: Smoked Salmon and Avocado Toast

- Lunch: Turkey and Hummus Wrap

- Dinner: Quinoa Stuffed Bell Peppers

- Dessert: Coconut Mango Rice Pudding

Day 7:

- Breakfast: Berry and Almond Butter Smoothie

- Lunch: Veggie Stir-Fry with Tofu

- Dinner: Lentil and Vegetable Soup

- Dessert: Almond Butter and Banana Ice Cream

Day 8:

- Breakfast: Avocado and Egg Breakfast Bowl

- Lunch: Mediterranean Chickpea Salad

- Dinner: Baked Lemon Herb Chicken

- Dessert: Berry and Yogurt Popsicles

Day 9:

- Breakfast: Greek Yogurt Parfait

- Lunch: Grilled Chicken and Vegetable Skewers

- Dinner: Lentil and Vegetable Soup

- Dessert: Banana and Peanut Butter Bites

Day 10:

- Breakfast: Spinach and Feta Omelette

- Lunch: Quinoa and Black Bean Stuffed Bell Peppers

- Dinner: Shrimp and Vegetable Stir-Fry

- Dessert: Greek Yogurt with Berries

Day 11:

- Breakfast: Quinoa Breakfast Bowl

- Lunch: Salmon and Asparagus Foil Packets

- Dinner: Turkey and Vegetable Skillet

- Dessert: Chia Seed Pudding with Mango

Day 12:

- Breakfast: Chia Seed Pudding

- Lunch: Eggplant Parmesan

- Dinner: Baked Salmon with Roasted Vegetables

- Dessert: Baked Pear with Almonds

Day 13:

- Breakfast: Smoked Salmon and Avocado Toast

- Lunch: Turkey and Hummus Wrap

- Dinner: Quinoa Stuffed Bell Peppers

- Dessert: Coconut Mango Rice Pudding

Day 14:

- Breakfast: Berry and Almond Butter Smoothie

- Lunch: Veggie Stir-Fry with Tofu

- Dinner: Lentil and Vegetable Soup

- Dessert: Almond Butter and Banana Ice Cream

Day 15:

- Breakfast: Avocado and Egg Breakfast Bowl

- Lunch: Mediterranean Chickpea Salad

- Dinner: Baked Lemon Herb Chicken

- Dessert: Baked Apple with Cinnamon

Day 16:

- Breakfast: Greek Yogurt Parfait

- Lunch: Grilled Chicken and Vegetable Skewers

- Dinner: Lentil and Vegetable Soup

- Dessert: Banana and Peanut Butter Bites

Day 17:

- Breakfast: Spinach and Feta Omelette

- Lunch: Quinoa and Black Bean Stuffed Bell Peppers

- Dinner: Shrimp and Vegetable Stir-Fry

- Dessert: Greek Yogurt with Berries

Day 18:

- Breakfast: Quinoa Breakfast Bowl

- Lunch: Salmon and Asparagus Foil Packets

- Dinner: Turkey and Vegetable Skillet

- Dessert: Chia Seed Pudding with Mango

Day 19:

- Breakfast: Chia Seed Pudding

- Lunch: Eggplant Parmesan

- Dinner: Baked Salmon with Roasted Vegetables

- Dessert: Baked Pear with Almonds

Day 20:

- Breakfast: Smoked Salmon and Avocado Toast

- Lunch: Turkey and Hummus Wrap

- Dinner: Quinoa Stuffed Bell Peppers

- Dessert: Coconut Mango Rice Pudding

Day 21:

- Breakfast: Berry and Almond Butter Smoothie

- Lunch: Veggie Stir-Fry with Tofu

- Dinner: Lentil and Vegetable Soup

- Dessert: Almond Butter and Banana Ice Cream

Day 22:

- Breakfast: Avocado and Egg Breakfast Bowl

- Lunch: Mediterranean Chickpea Salad

- Dinner: Baked Lemon Herb Chicken

- Dessert: Berry and Yogurt Popsicles

Day 23:

- Breakfast: Greek Yogurt Parfait

- Lunch: Grilled Chicken and Vegetable Skewers

- Dinner: Lentil and Vegetable Soup

- Dessert: Banana and Peanut Butter Bites

Day 24:

- Breakfast: Spinach and Feta Omelette

- Lunch: Quinoa and Black Bean Stuffed Bell Peppers

- Dinner: Shrimp and Vegetable Stir-Fry

- Dessert: Greek Yogurt with Berries

Day 25:

- Breakfast: Quinoa Breakfast Bowl

- Lunch: Salmon and Asparagus Foil Packets

- Dinner: Turkey and Vegetable Skillet

- Dessert: Chia Seed Pudding with Mango

Day 26:

- Breakfast: Chia Seed Pudding

- Lunch: Eggplant Parmesan

- Dinner: Baked Salmon with Roasted Vegetables

- Dessert: Baked Pear with Almonds

Day 27:

- Breakfast: Smoked Salmon and Avocado Toast

- Lunch: Turkey and Hummus Wrap

- Dinner: Quinoa Stuffed Bell Peppers

- Dessert: Coconut Mango Rice Pudding

Day 28:

- Breakfast: Berry and Almond Butter Smoothie

- Lunch: Veggie Stir-Fry with Tofu

- Dinner: Lentil and Vegetable Soup

- Dessert: Almond Butter and Banana Ice Cream

CHAPTER 7

EXERCISE AND PHYSICAL ACTIVITY

In the symphony of senior health, exercise and physical activity compose the vibrant melody that uplifts the spirit, fortifies the body, and enriches the journey of aging with vitality and resilience. Within the confines of this chapter, we shall embark on a journey into the heart of exercise for seniors, unraveling its profound importance and exploring a myriad of suitable types tailored to nurture the aging body and mind.

Importance of Exercise for Seniors

Picture a majestic oak tree, its sturdy trunk anchored firmly in the earth, its branches reaching skyward in a graceful dance with the wind. Much like this venerable tree, the human body thrives on movement – it is the essence of life itself, the elixir that sustains vitality and fortifies resilience in the face of time's gentle embrace.

For seniors, the importance of exercise transcends mere physicality; it is a cornerstone of holistic well-being that nourishes the body, mind, and spirit in equal measure. As the sands of time trickle down, our bodies undergo a series of changes that demand deliberate attention to movement and physical activity.

Physical activity serves as a potent elixir for aging bodies, bestowing upon them a wealth of benefits that extend far beyond the confines of muscle and bone. From bolstering cardiovascular health and improving balance to enhancing cognitive function and fostering emotional well-being, the transformative power of exercise knows no bounds.

Regular exercise has been shown to reduce the risk of chronic diseases such as heart disease, diabetes, and osteoporosis – formidable adversaries that often loom on the horizon as we age. Moreover, it serves as a potent ally in the battle against age-related cognitive decline, sharpening cognition, and preserving memory function well into the golden years.

But perhaps most importantly, exercise is the cornerstone of independence and vitality in senior life. By fostering strength, flexibility, and mobility, it empowers seniors to navigate the intricacies of daily life with grace and confidence, preserving their autonomy and dignity in the face of life's myriad challenges.

In essence, exercise is the fountain of youth that flows within us, waiting to be unleashed with each step, each stretch, each joyful movement. It is the gentle caress of vitality that breathes life into aging bodies, infusing them with the vibrancy and resilience to embrace each day with open arms.

Types of Exercise Suitable for Seniors

Now that we've established the profound importance of exercise for seniors, let's delve into the myriad of types tailored to meet the unique needs and preferences of aging bodies.

1. **Aerobic Exercise**: Also known as cardio, aerobic exercise encompasses activities that elevate the heart rate and increase oxygen consumption, thereby improving cardiovascular health. Suitable options for seniors include brisk walking, swimming, cycling, and dancing. These activities not only strengthen the heart and lungs but also enhance endurance and promote overall well-being.

2. **Strength Training**: Strength training, also referred to as resistance training, involves using resistance to build muscle strength and endurance. This type of exercise is particularly beneficial for seniors as it helps counteract age-related muscle loss and preserve bone density, reducing the risk of falls and fractures. Examples of

strength training exercises include lifting weights, using resistance bands, and performing bodyweight exercises such as squats, lunges, and push-ups.

3. **Flexibility and Balance Exercises**: Flexibility and balance exercises are essential for seniors to maintain mobility, prevent injuries, and enhance overall physical function. These exercises focus on improving range of motion, joint flexibility, and proprioception. Activities such as yoga, tai chi, and Pilates are excellent choices for seniors as they not only promote flexibility and balance but also foster relaxation and stress relief.

4. **Low-Impact Activities**: For seniors with joint issues or mobility limitations, low-impact activities provide an excellent alternative to high-impact exercises. These activities are gentle on the joints while still offering cardiovascular benefits. Examples include walking, water aerobics, stationary biking, and elliptical training.

5. **Functional Training**: Functional training focuses on exercises that mimic everyday movements, helping seniors maintain independence in activities of daily living. This type of exercise emphasizes movements that engage multiple muscle groups and improve coordination, stability, and mobility. Examples include

squats, lunges, step-ups, and functional resistance exercises using resistance bands or cable machines.

6. **Mind-Body Exercises**: Mind-body exercises such as yoga, tai chi, and qigong offer a holistic approach to fitness that integrates physical movement with mental focus and relaxation techniques. These practices not only improve flexibility, balance, and strength but also promote mindfulness, stress reduction, and emotional well-being.

CHAPTER 8

TIPS FOR SUCCESSFUL IMPLEMENTATION

In the journey toward adopting a metabolic reset diet, the path of transition is paved with intention, mindfulness, and a steadfast commitment to nurturing your body's innate wisdom. As we embark on this transformative odyssey, let us navigate the waters of change with grace, embracing the gentle rhythm of gradual transition that honors our body's unique needs and rhythms.

The Importance of Gradual Transition

Imagine embarking on a journey into uncharted territory without a compass or a map. The terrain ahead may seem daunting, filled with unfamiliar twists and turns that leave you feeling overwhelmed and disoriented. This analogy holds true when embarking on a metabolic reset diet. Transitioning abruptly from your current eating habits to a radically different dietary approach can shock your system and trigger a cascade of physical and emotional reactions.

Enter the concept of gradual transition—a guiding principle that emphasizes the importance of easing into a new way of eating with patience, mindfulness, and a deep sense of self-awareness. By taking small, deliberate steps toward change, you give your body the time it needs to adjust, adapt, and thrive.

Setting Realistic Goals

Before diving headfirst into the waters of change, take a moment to set realistic goals that reflect your unique needs, preferences, and lifestyle. Whether your aim is to shed excess weight, boost your energy levels, or improve your overall health, framing your goals in a clear, concrete manner sets the stage for success.

Remember, Rome wasn't built in a day, and neither will your metabolic reset journey unfold overnight. Be gentle with yourself, celebrate small victories along the way, and embrace the journey as an opportunity for growth, learning, and self-discovery.

Seeking Professional Guidance

In the vast landscape of dietary approaches, navigating the terrain can feel overwhelming, especially for those embarking on their first metabolic reset journey. This is where seeking professional guidance can make all the difference.

Consider consulting with a registered dietitian or nutritionist who specializes in senior health and metabolic wellness. These professionals possess the expertise, knowledge, and experience to tailor a metabolic reset plan that aligns with your unique needs, preferences, and health goals.

During your consultation, be open and honest about your current eating habits, medical history, and any specific dietary restrictions or preferences you may have. Together, you and your nutrition expert can co-create a personalized roadmap for success, complete with practical strategies, meal plans, and lifestyle recommendations to support your metabolic reset journey.

Remember, you don't have to navigate this journey alone. With the guidance of a qualified professional by your side, you can embark on your metabolic reset journey with confidence, clarity, and peace of mind.

Tracking Progress

As the saying goes, "What gets measured gets managed." In the realm of metabolic reset diets, tracking your progress is an invaluable tool for staying accountable, monitoring your success, and making informed adjustments along the way.

Consider keeping a food journal to record your daily meals, snacks, and fluid intake. This simple yet powerful practice not only heightens your awareness of your eating habits but also provides valuable insights into patterns, triggers, and areas for improvement.

In addition to tracking your food intake, pay attention to how your body responds to the changes you're making. Are you noticing improvements in your energy levels, mood, and overall well-being? Are you experiencing any unexpected challenges or setbacks? By staying attuned to your body's signals and feedback, you can fine-tune your metabolic reset plan to better suit your evolving needs.

Moreover, don't underestimate the power of non-scale victories. While weight loss may be a common goal of metabolic reset diets, it's essential to celebrate other signs of progress, such as improved sleep quality, enhanced mental clarity, and increased vitality.

CHAPTER 9

POTENTIAL CHALLENGES AND HOW TO OVERCOME THEM

Embarking on a metabolic reset diet journey for seniors is a commendable endeavor, but like any path to wellness, it's not without its hurdles. In this chapter, we'll delve into the potential challenges that may arise along the way and explore effective strategies for overcoming them.

Social Situations

Navigating social situations while adhering to a metabolic reset diet can present its own set of challenges. Whether it's family gatherings, dinner parties, or outings with friends, food often takes center stage in social interactions. Here's how to tackle these situations with grace and confidence:

1. **Communication is Key**: Don't be afraid to communicate your dietary preferences and goals to friends and family. Let them know that you're following a metabolic reset diet for health reasons and kindly request their support in making meal choices that align with your plan.

2. **Plan Ahead**: If you know you'll be attending a social event where food choices may be limited, consider

eating a balanced meal beforehand to curb hunger and temptation. Additionally, bring along a nutritious snack or dish to share, ensuring you have a healthy option available.

3. **Focus on Connections**: Shift the focus of social gatherings away from food and towards meaningful connections with loved ones. Engage in conversation, participate in activities, and enjoy the company of those around you, reminding yourself that nourishment comes in many forms beyond what's on your plate.

4. **Flexibility is Key**: While it's important to stay committed to your metabolic reset diet, it's also essential to be flexible when necessary. If you find yourself in a situation where adhering strictly to your plan is challenging, aim for moderation and make the best choices available without feeling guilty.

5. **Mindful Eating**: Practice mindful eating during social gatherings by paying attention to hunger and fullness cues, savoring each bite, and making intentional choices that support your health goals.

Overcoming Cravings

Cravings can be a formidable adversary on the journey to metabolic reset, but armed with the right strategies, you can conquer them and stay on track with your dietary goals. Here's how to tackle cravings head-on:

1. **Identify Triggers**: Pay attention to the triggers that prompt cravings, whether it's stress, emotions, or environmental cues. By identifying these triggers, you can develop strategies to address them effectively.

2. **Stay Hydrated**: Sometimes, thirst can masquerade as hunger, leading to unnecessary cravings. Stay hydrated by drinking plenty of water throughout the day, especially before meals and when cravings strike.

3. **Opt for Nutrient-Dense Foods**: Choose nutrient-dense foods that satisfy cravings while supporting your metabolic reset goals. For example, if you're craving something sweet, opt for fruits like berries or a small piece of dark chocolate instead of sugary treats.

4. **Practice Mindful Eating**: Slow down and savor each bite when eating, paying attention to the taste, texture, and satisfaction derived from food. By practicing mindful eating, you can better tune into your body's hunger and fullness signals, reducing the likelihood of succumbing to cravings.

5. **Distract Yourself**: Engage in activities that distract you from cravings, whether it's going for a walk, practicing a

hobby, or engaging in a conversation with a friend. By shifting your focus away from food, you can diminish the intensity of cravings and redirect your energy towards more productive pursuits.

Dealing with Plateaus

Plateaus are a common occurrence in any dietary journey, including metabolic reset diets. These periods of stagnant progress can be frustrating, but they also present an opportunity for reflection and adjustment. Here's how to navigate plateaus with resilience and determination:

1. **Reassess Your Plan**: Take a step back and reassess your metabolic reset plan, including your dietary choices, exercise routine, and lifestyle factors. Are there any areas where you could make improvements or adjustments? Consider consulting with a healthcare professional or nutritionist for personalized guidance.

2. **Mix Up Your Routine**: Plateaus can sometimes be broken by introducing variety into your routine. Try incorporating new foods, recipes, or exercise activities to stimulate your metabolism and reignite progress.

3. **Stay Consistent**: Consistency is key when it comes to overcoming plateaus. Stay committed to your metabolic

reset plan, even when progress seems slow or non-existent. Trust the process and remain patient, knowing that small, consistent efforts will eventually yield results.

4. **Focus on Non-Scale Victories**: Instead of solely focusing on the number on the scale, celebrate non-scale victories such as increased energy levels, improved mood, or enhanced physical fitness. These indicators of progress are just as important, if not more so, than changes in weight.

5. **Practice Self-Compassion**: Be kind to yourself during plateaus and avoid self-criticism or negative self-talk. Remember that setbacks are a natural part of any journey, and what's important is how you respond to them. Treat yourself with compassion, patience, and resilience as you navigate through challenging times.

CHAPTER 10

PRECAUTIONS AND CONSIDERATIONS

As we delve deeper into the realm of metabolic reset diets for seniors, it's crucial to tread carefully and mindfully. While the benefits of such dietary interventions are vast and promising, it's equally important to navigate potential pitfalls with wisdom and caution. In this chapter, we'll explore a trifecta of precautions and considerations: consulting a healthcare professional, managing medications, and adapting for individual needs.

Consulting a Healthcare Professional

Before embarking on any dietary journey, especially one as transformative as a metabolic reset diet, it's essential to seek guidance from a qualified healthcare professional. This could be your primary care physician, a registered dietitian, or a nutritionist specializing in senior health.

Why is consulting a healthcare professional so crucial? Firstly, they can assess your current health status and provide personalized recommendations tailored to your unique needs and medical history. They can help you navigate any underlying health conditions or dietary restrictions that may impact your ability to adhere to a metabolic reset diet safely.

Moreover, healthcare professionals serve as invaluable allies on your journey toward better health. They can monitor your progress, address any concerns or challenges that arise, and make adjustments to your dietary plan as needed. By forging a collaborative partnership with your healthcare team, you empower yourself to make informed decisions that support your overall well-being.

So, before you take the plunge into the waters of metabolic reset diets, schedule a consultation with your healthcare professional. Together, you can chart a course toward vibrant health and vitality that's rooted in knowledge, support, and expert guidance.

Managing Medications

For many seniors, managing medications is a daily reality that cannot be overlooked when embarking on a metabolic reset diet. Prescription medications, over-the-counter supplements, and herbal remedies may all play a role in your health regimen, and it's essential to navigate their interactions with dietary changes with caution and foresight.

One crucial consideration is the potential impact of dietary modifications on medication efficacy and absorption. Some foods and nutrients may interact with certain medications, either enhancing or inhibiting their effects. For example, grapefruit juice can interfere with the metabolism of certain medications, while high-fiber foods may affect the absorption of others.

Additionally, drastic changes in diet, such as sudden shifts in macronutrient ratios or calorie intake, can impact blood sugar levels, blood pressure, and other physiological parameters that may influence medication dosages. This underscores the importance of regular monitoring and communication with your healthcare provider to ensure that your medication regimen remains safe and effective throughout your dietary journey.

Furthermore, certain dietary supplements and herbal remedies may interact with medications, either amplifying or counteracting their effects. It's crucial to disclose all supplements and alternative remedies you're taking to your healthcare provider to avoid potential complications or adverse reactions.

CONCLUSION

n the vast tapestry of dietary interventions, the metabolic reset diet for seniors emerges as a beacon of hope and possibility, offering a transformative journey toward vitality, longevity, and holistic well-being. As we draw the curtains on this exploration of rejuvenating metabolic health in the golden years, let us pause to reflect on the key points illuminated along the way and the profound long-term benefits that await those who dare to embark on this path of renewal.

Recap of Key Points

Throughout our journey, we've delved into the intricacies of metabolic reset diets for seniors, unraveling the tapestry of principles, strategies, and considerations that underpin this transformative approach to health:

1. **Understanding Metabolism**: We've explored the intricate dance of biochemical processes that govern metabolism, and the profound impact of aging on its rhythm and tempo.

2. **Principles of Metabolic Reset Diet**: We've embraced the principles of balance, nourishment, and sustainability, recognizing the power of whole foods,

balanced macronutrients, and mindful hydration in recalibrating metabolism.

3. **Benefits for Seniors**: We've witnessed the myriad benefits that await those who embrace a metabolic reset diet, from weight management and energy restoration to cognitive clarity and disease prevention.

4. **Key Components**: We've navigated the terrain of dietary components, from the importance of whole foods and fiber to the nuances of portion control and meal planning.

5. **Exercise and Physical Activity**: We've acknowledged the synergistic relationship between diet and exercise, recognizing the importance of physical activity in supporting metabolic health and overall well-being.

6. **Tips for Success**: We've armed ourselves with practical strategies for success, from gradual transition and professional guidance to tracking progress and overcoming challenges.

7. **Precautions and Considerations**: We've heeded the call for caution and mindfulness, recognizing the importance of consulting healthcare professionals, managing medications, and adapting dietary plans to individual needs.

Long-Term Benefits of Metabolic Reset Diet for Seniors

As we bid farewell to the shores of exploration and venture into the horizon of possibility, let us cast our gaze toward the long-term benefits that await those who embrace the transformative power of metabolic reset diets for seniors:

1. **Vitality and Energy**: By recalibrating metabolism and fueling the body with nutrient-dense foods, seniors can experience renewed vitality, sustained energy levels, and a zest for life that defies the passage of time.

2. **Health and Wellness**: Through the synergistic interplay of balanced nutrition, regular exercise, and mindful lifestyle choices, seniors can mitigate the risk of chronic diseases, support immune function, and foster overall wellness that transcends mere physical health.

3. **Cognitive Clarity**: Nourishing the brain with essential nutrients and supporting cognitive function through dietary interventions can lead to improved memory, sharper cognition, and enhanced mental clarity that enriches daily life and fosters a sense of empowerment and independence.

4. **Quality of Life**: Ultimately, the true measure of success lies not just in the absence of disease but in the

presence of vibrant health, joy, and fulfillment. By embracing a metabolic reset diet, seniors can reclaim control of their health destiny, savoring each moment and embracing the journey of aging with grace, resilience, and unwavering vitality.

In conclusion, the metabolic reset diet for seniors offers a gateway to a future brimming with possibility and promise. By embracing the principles of balance, nourishment, and mindfulness, and by navigating the terrain of dietary exploration with wisdom and intention, seniors can unlock the door to a life rich in vitality, wellness, and joy. So, let us embark on this odyssey of transformation together, as we harness the power of metabolic reset diets to sculpt a future filled with health, happiness, and boundless potential.

www.ingramcontent.com/pod-product-compliance
Lightning Source LLC
Chambersburg PA
CBHW070823260726

48660CB00005B/1964